The Little Book of Laughnosis

*Using the Hypnotic Power
of Unconditional Laughter
to Change Lives*

by
James Hazlerig, MA

Foreword by
Dave Berman, ChT

Copyright © 2016 by James A. Hazlerig

All rights reserved. This book or any portion thereof may not be reproduced or used in any manner whatsoever without the express written permission of the publisher except for the use of brief quotations in a book review.

Table of Contents

FOREWORD i
LAUGHNOSIS FOUND 1
    An Epidemic of Seriosity 3
    SLEEP! Or Better Yet, LAUGH! 5
    Nota Bene: What to Do if Your Hypnotic Subject Starts Laughing 10
    Hebb's Law, or How Laughter Can Change Your Brain 11
    Objections to Laughnosis 16
EXERCISES 20
    Exercise One: Stress Ball with Laughter 22
    Exercise Two: Laughter Bubble Plus 26
    Exercise Three: Bi-LAUGHTER-al Stimulation 28
    Exercise Four: Laughter-Mations 31
    Exercise Five: Body-Positive Laughter-Mations 33
    Exercise Six: Laughter as an Auditory Submodality Shift 35
    Exercise Seven: Riddikulus Charm / Laughter Swish 37
    Exercise Eight: Laughter Re-Programming 39
    Exercise Nine: Laughter Re-Programming for Procrastination 42
    Becoming Laughnotic 44
FINAL WORDS 50
    Shoulders of Giants 51
    References 53
    Further Action 54

FOREWORD

James Hazlerig and I first met in Redondo Beach, California, when Scott Sandland and Richard Clark convened the inaugural class of the Hypnosis Practitioner Training Institute in January 2012. As I read *The Little Book of Laughnosis*, I caught glimpses of the influence we both absorbed in that next year of study together. In particular, by the time I got to page 41, I was anticipating James's reference to "being hypnotic" and was already mentally writing this Foreword about it.

You see, we were taught a conceptual understanding of hypnosis that transcends memorization of mechanical steps to take. It was presented to us as analogous to becoming a chef capable of improvising a gourmet meal with last minute surprise ingredients rather than being a cook capable only of following a recipe.

The Little Book of Laughnosis offers a similar approach to understanding and utilizing the benefits of laughing on purpose. That means as you read this book you will get both specific instructions you can follow and general ideas you can extrapolate. I recommend you start with this one formulated in a classic hypnotic language pattern:

The more you laugh on purpose, the more life shows you reasons to laugh.

This may just be the antidote to the seriosity epidemic James describes because you will feel good whether your laughter is triggered by external stimuli or generated by choice from within. And as you develop your practice of voluntary laughter you will likely find you meet the irritating or even mundane moments of your life with a new perspective and response.

The central premise of *Laughter For the Health of It,* the book I co-wrote with fellow hypnotist Kelley T. Woods, is the mind/body principles that make hypnosis work are the same ones responsible for the physiological, psychological, neurological, and chemical changes that occur from laughing. More specifically, in hypnosis we say the body can't tell the difference between responding to something real or vividly imagined. In Laughter Yoga we say the body can't tell the difference between laughing at something funny ("conditional" laughter) and laughing intentionally ("unconditional" laughter).

James takes our thesis a step further, illustrating how the basic hypnotic principle of bypassing the conscious mind to reach the subconscious is also achieved by laughter. The best part is you don't even have to be funny or learn to remember a bunch of jokes. If you understand the idea of "being hypnotic," then you can get on board with what James calls being "laughnotic."

Just as hypnotists learn we must "go there first," we must also be able to generate spontaneous laughter if we are to introduce it to our clients. As you read on, James will share with you some of his personal laughter hygiene, or how he incorporates intentional laughter into his own self-care and wellness. I invite you to consider this a starting point in cultivating your own daily laughter practice.

Inspiring people to become Daily Laughers has become a personal mission for me. Every day in 2016 I produce a new video demonstrating different ways to laugh on purpose. Some of the videos show me laughing alone but most include a guest. By the end of the year I will have laughed with people in all 50 United States and at least 50 other countries. This work resulted in Laughter Yoga Co-Founders Dr. Madan Kataria and Madhuri Kataria honoring me with the designation of Laughter Ambassador.

Laughter is a Universal language that can be communicated without words to bond us socially or therapeutically on the strength of the neurotransmitter oxytocin. Laughing every day will allow you to accrue benefits beyond the immediate joyfulness and stress reduction, including boosting your immune system, improving circulation, increasing pain tolerance, and evolving your world view to include more playfulness, mindfulness, creativity, and acceptance of others.

These health, social, and spiritual benefits are available to all who choose to tap into them via laughter. By their nature, these life enhancements will impact the people in your life. Therefore, in my view, the Daily Laughers YouTube channel is a pebble in a pond, making ripple effects outward to an ultimate impact beyond what we can imagine now. It is no mystery, however, that the intention is aligned with Dr. Kataria's mission of creating world peace through laughter.

Allow that to start from within you, laughing on purpose each and every day.

Dave Berman, C.Ht.
Laughter Ambassador, Hypnotherapist, Coach, Speaker & Author
http://DailyLaughers.com
http://ManifestPositivity.com

LAUGHNOSIS FOUND

An Epidemic of Seriosity

A severe, unrecognized, undiagnosed epidemic is burning in our society.

I see the victims everyday. They trudge into my hypnosis office, their heads hanging low, shoulders drooping, breath unnaturally shallow. I see this epidemic in the dour expressions of some of the psychologists and counsellors with whom I share a waiting room. Some suffer so severely they cannot muster a smile of greeting. I see it in the angry faces of fellow motorists on the freeway, driving as though they wish everyone else would just get out of their way — maneuvering, honking, cursing, and gesturing as though a few seconds' advantage on a daily commute were some sort of evolutionary imperative. And, I must confess, I have seen myself relapse whenever I forget to take preventative measures.

It is an Epidemic of Seriosity.

Seriosity, also known as Excessive Seriousness, Grumpypants-Frownyface Syndrome, and/or Acute Laughter and Fun Deficiency is a neurological disorder in which brain pathways that support healthy emotional and immune responses have atrophied due to disuse, while neural pathways leading to unhealthy thoughts, emotions, and behaviors have become stronger and stronger over time. It operates as a feedback loop: The worse you feel, the grumpier you get; the grumpier you get, the worse you feel.

At the end of all my hypnosis sessions, I ask my clients to look to their left, where I have a small yellow smiley-face attached to the wall. When they press it at my request, the Emergency Affirmation button makes a sound like a harp, followed by the unbelievably enthusiastic words, "YOU ARE AWESOME!" This inevitably gets a laugh.

Not long ago, I had just finished a session helping a lovely older lady release the grief she felt when her dog died. After hitting the button, she laughed uproariously and then said, "Oh! It's been so long since I laughed!" When I asked how long she meant, she replied, "Months—nearly a year!"

There it was—Intense Chronic Seriosity.

Fortunately, there is an antidote for Seriosity, a way to reverse its effects. There is a method to re-route those negative brain pathways, employing self-directed neuroplasticity, to lead us into healthier, happier, more blissful emotional responses.

The antidote to Seriosity is Laughnosis.

This short book will teach you simple, practical ways to change your life and the lives of those around you.

SLEEP! Or Better Yet, LAUGH!

To understand Laughnosis, you'll need a basic understanding of hypnosis. (On the other hand, to use Laughnosis, you don't need to know how it works. Feel free to skip right to the exercises and start feeling better and changing your life immediately.)

But back to hypnosis. Now, before your mind runs away with bizarre notions of spinning spirals, swinging pocket watches, and hapless victims clucking like chickens, let me just say that hypnosis is NOT what you've seen on TV or in the movies.

Many people believe it's a state of trance or relaxation. While both of those can happen with hypnosis, for our purposes in this book, I'm going to drop that part of the definition and instead focus on a phrase commonly used in hypnosis definitions:

"Bypass of the Critical Faculty"

See, whether they define hypnosis as some kind of trance state or view it as a process and interaction, most hypnotists agree that in some way, we bypass or nullify that part of the mind that fact-checks, that part of the mind that questions new ideas to decide whether they'll be accepted as true. Though it's a term with slightly archaic origins, we call that part of the mind the "critical faculty." Getting past it in order to make effective suggestions is really what hypnosis is all about.

To give you a few examples, when you go to a movie, watch TV, or read a good book, chances are that you bypass your critical faculty (also known as "suspending disbelief"). If you are engaged in a sad story, you might feel real sadness and shed real tears, even though you know that the story is completely made up, the characters are just actors, and the dog didn't really die. The part of your mind that would normally be busily reminding you that it's all imaginary has taken a break, leaving you ready to accept suggestions and experience real reactions to imaginary events.

Another very clear example is worry. Far too many people dwell on hypothetical disasters, imagining misfortunes to such a degree that their bodies and brains literally go into fight or flight mode, as though they were being attacked or physically threatened. Sometimes it's that low-level stress that seems to play in the background of life, and other times it can be a full-blown panic attack. In either case, the critical faculty has been bypassed, and real physiological results arise from imaginary events.

Of course, the more dramatic version of this is what you may have seen in hypnosis stage shows, when people who are particularly good at shutting off their critical faculties and engaging their imaginations begin to react to every made-up situation as though it were real, accepting every suggestion as though it were truth.

Now, the interesting connection between laughter and hypnosis is this:

Laughter Bypasses the Critical Faculty.

Evidence for this fact shows up in several interesting psychological studies. In the first of these, volunteers were asked to read jokes into a microphone, ostensibly for a study on how vocal intonation affects humor. One group was asked to read jokes that disparaged people from a particular region—Newfoundland. The control group read jokes of a neutral nature. Afterwards, all participants were asked their opinions of "Newfies." The first group, exposed to the bigoted jabs, expressed low opinions of the Newfoundlanders, having been influenced by the jokes.

In an even more alarming study, women of all hair colors were divided into two groups. One group read "blonde jokes" into a microphone for an hour, while the rest did not. All were then given an intelligence test. The blonde women who had spent an hour reading jokes that suggested they were stupid scored significantly lower than their fair-haired counterparts who had not read the disparaging jokes.

I've had my own experience with this as well. When I was eighteen, I passed out shortly after giving blood; a few months later, I passed out while attempting to poke my finger in biology lab. After that, any time I had to give blood, I would light-heartedly say, "You'd better lie me down; my body doesn't like to give up its blood." I did this for well over a decade.

Eventually, though, I decided to donate blood again. I made my usual joke, and the phlebotomists at the blood center accommodatingly let me lie down. The first technician tried twice to get my blood before calling her supervisor, who stuck me three times before getting only enough blood to fill the tube. She asked me to squeeze a ball, to move my hand in different ways, to take deep breaths—nothing changed the outcome. Throughout the ordeal, I kept making my joke about my body not wanting to give up its blood.

Well, I wasn't yet a hypnotist, but I had been reading at the time about the power of suggestion, and I realized suddenly that by making that joke repeatedly, I was in fact engaging in self-suggestion. Could I actually be preventing my blood from flowing into the tube? To test that theory, I visualized a cartoon in which my blood flowed through the needle and tube, all the way into the receptacle. At that moment, the phlebotomist shouted, "Whatever you're doing, keep doing it!"

Jokes, by their nature, are not taken seriously; in other words, they aren't fact-checked. They bypass the critical faculty and take on the power of hypnotic suggestions, especially when repeated. (Repetition is another method for bypassing the critical faculty.)

Acting As-If

Another way to bypass the critical faculty is to act as-if something were true. This is popularly known as "faking it 'till you make it."

For example, one popular hypnotic technique for working with "resistant" clients is to say, "Science shows that you can actually get all the benefits of hypnosis without being hypnotized, if you simply pretend that you are deeply hypnotized. So as I say these words, act as if you were the most hypnotizable person in the world and respond accordingly." This inevitably leads to a bypass of the critical faculty, often resulting in trance as well.

Most hypnosis stage shows start out with asking volunteers to pretend they are auditioning for a movie, and the role will require them to act as though they were seeing something very funny. The volunteers are then encouraged to laugh their heads off. (Appearing sad, scared, hot, and/or cold often complete this routine.) Interestingly, most volunteers soon begin to actually feel euphoric, sad, scared, hot and/or cold even though they were merely instructed to act as if they were feeling that way. Though not officially part of the hypnotic induction, this phase of a show is an important part of the hypnotic process.

This of course ties into the psycho-physiological principle that emotion follows motion. In other words, we don't laugh because we're happy; we're happy because we laugh. As Dr. Madan Kataria points out in his Laughter Yoga teachings, your body doesn't know the difference between spontaneous, Conditional Laughter and forced, Unconditional Laughter. Your body experiences the same enhanced oxygenation from both, and your brain generates the same wonderful, feel-good neurotransmitters in either case: endorphins, dopamine, serotonin, and oxytocin.

The principle that laughing bypasses the critical faculty and therefore increases suggestibility, though not emphasized in the Laughter Yoga training materials, is mentioned in passing.

Nota Bene: What to Do if Your Hypnotic Subject Starts Laughing

Back when I was a fairly new hypnotist, I was working with a teenaged girl. Going through a progressive muscle relaxation, I suggested that each part of her body relax: her feet, her calves, her knees, her thighs, her buttocks …

She burst out laughing at that point.

Let's face it, "buttocks" is a pretty funny sounding word. (I've since borrowed terminology from equestrians, so I refer to the "muscles of the seat.")

The problem was that she wouldn't stop laughing. Now, many hypnotists would simply end the session or get angry that the subject wasn't taking things seriously. However, remembering the principles of Milton Erickson, I utilized her laughter: "That's right—buttocks is a hilarious word, and you're right to laugh. In fact, the more you laugh, the better you feel, and the better you feel, the deeper you go. Have you ever been in a place where you weren't supposed to laugh—like a library or a wedding—and you just couldn't stop? Just when you would almost stop, you'd think, BUTTOCKS! And you'd laugh again."

So I guided her through her laughter until it subsided, interspersing suggestions for our goal the whole time.

Hebb's Law,
or How Laughter Can Change Your Brain

In 1949, neuro-psychologist Donald Hebb published *The Organization of Behavior,* in which he stated a foundational principle of neuro-science that happens to also provide a physical basis for all hypnotic changework:

"Neurons that fire together, wire together."

In other words, any time you think a thought, feel a feeling, or perform an action, the mental pathway of neurons associated with that thought, feeling, or action becomes stronger. I like to explain it to my clients using this metaphor:

The first time you walk through a forest, it's a lot of work. You have to take out a machete and hack your way through, carefully plotting your course and watching your footing. The next day, it's much easier, but you still have to trim some plants out of the way. The next time you walk the path, you might remove some of the worst rocks, and so on, working to widen the path each day. Eventually, it's no effort at all, and then at some point after that, the path starts to become a groove, and we all know how easy something is once we find our groove.

The only problem comes if we realize we don't like where the path is going, but the groove makes it so easy to go there without any effort or conscious thought. In fact, that's when the groove becomes a rut, and we get stuck in negative self-talk (aka "stinkin' thinkin'") and harmful behaviors that seem automatic.

Fortunately, Hebb's Law has a corollary that provides us with hope:

"Neurons that fire out of sync, lose their link."

In other words, if a pattern is interrupted and the thoughts scrambled, then the connection between stimulus and response is weakened. It's as though we've put up a roadblock and bulldozed part of the original path, letting the rest get overgrown with weeds.

Many of the interventions used in modern hypnosis and Neuro-Linguistic Programming (NLP) are based on Hebb's Principles, popularly known as neuroplasticity. Pavlov's discoveries about conditioning stimulus and response are also important here.

One such intervention is an NLP method called "The Swish Pattern." It basically involves picturing a trigger that usually inspires some undesirable response (such as a red traffic light, which may stimulate frustration and anger) and then replacing it with a desirable response (such as smiling, laughing, and remaining calm in traffic). When repeated enough times very quickly, this technique can link the old stimulus to the new, desired response in such a way that stopping at a red light elicits smiles, laughter, and calmness rather than frustration and anger. On a neurological level, the brain is "re-wired"; in a sense, one becomes a whole new person.

Now as Carson and Marion point out in their highly-recommended book, *The Swish: An In Depth Look at this Powerful NLP Pattern,* the mind can be considered an engine for classifying things into groups. As a result, several Swish Patterns with similar stimuli all tying to the same response will often produce generative change. For example, in the case above, linking several aggravating traffic situations to smiling, laughing, and remaining calm establishes a kind of generalized connection between formerly frustrating traffic conditions and a more positive, amused response.

So what does all of this have to do with Laughter Yoga?

Well, there's a class of Laughter Yoga activities referred to as "value-based exercises." In each of these, participants pantomime (and to some degree visualize) unpleasant or frustrating situations while laughing in some way. In the "Look at My Bills" exercise, participants pantomime opening up imaginary bills and "laugh/weep" while pointing to the amount owed. In a group, each person shows the amount to the other members who laugh/weep in sympathy. (This exercise is often followed by the "Winning Lottery Ticket" exercise, in which participants celebrate winning an imaginary lottery.)

Another value-based exercise is "Red Light/Green Light," in which the laughter leader shouts "Green Light" to signal participants to pantomime zipping around the room in imaginary cars (making "vroom-vroom" noises) until the leader shouts, "Red Light," whereupon participants stop where they are and laugh uproariously until the leader shouts "Green Light" again.

While these exercises are outrageously fun and playful, the real benefits come later, when participants discover themselves laughing at actual red lights and other things that used to frustrate them in traffic, or feeling less alarmed and discouraged when confronted with a large bill to pay.

Essentially, value-based laughter exercises operate as a form of Swish Pattern, attaching a new response (laughter) to an old stimulus, creating new neural pathways that guide people toward better, happier responses. This is the essence of Laughnosis.

I have seen first-hand how these exercises lead to generative change, making laughter and amusement become the new default responses to situations that in many people lead to anger. Let me provide an example:

Several years ago, I shared a hotel room in Vegas with several of my fellow hypnotists, including Laughter Ambassador Dave Berman. Although I had been in Vegas for several days, he and our other room-mate had arrived at about three o'clock in the morning, having driven from California. At six that morning — which I should note was eight a.m. back at my home in the Great and Sovereign State of Texas — my alarm went off, blasting a very lively and slightly obnoxious hymn to Ganesh, sung in Hindi.

Now, I don't know about you, but if I've had only three hours' sleep, and I hear an alarm of any sort, much less someone else's idea of fun wake-up music, I am a bear. And not a fun, cuddly, heart-on-my-belly bear who cares about you; I'm talking a mean, growling, eager-to-rip-your-arm-off-unless-propitiated-with-very-strong-coffee kind of bear.

So that morning, as my alarm was blaring and my brain was still trying to sort out the meaning of it, I heard another sound along with it. The sound made no sense at first, and then I realized it was laughter. As my morning brain-fog slowly lifted, I realized that Dave—who'd had only three hours of sleep after a long drive—was laughing enthusiastically! When I asked him what was funny, he said that the music and situation were just so ridiculous that laughing was the only reasonable reaction.

I realized then and there that laughter had become his default response to things that would normally make me—and let's face it, a lot of people—annoyed, angry, or frustrated. The value-based exercises of Laughter Yoga, each one acting like its own Swish Pattern, had re-wired his brain and re-trained his mind to produce generative, positive change.

I also resolved, then and there, to learn how to use laughter to change myself and my clients for the better.

Objections to Laughnosis

In using and discussing the practices described in this book, I've encountered (and countered) a few objections from clients and fellow practitioners. Here's how I handle them.

As I mentioned before, many of my clients have Intense Chronic Seriosity. They haven't had a reason to smile or laugh — or at least not a reason they recognized as sufficient — so they've done neither for a long time, severely depriving their brains of endorphins, dopamine, serotonin, and oxytocin. They often describe themselves as full of depression and despair. Hebb's Laws have worked against them, deepening the ruts of hopelessness and humorlessness.

When guiding such clients through Laughnosis exercises, I find some object to smiling intentionally, saying, "It feels fake." See, they are laboring under the common delusions that our facial expressions arise from our emotions, and that it never works the other way around.

So I typically say, "Of course, it feels strange! You're doing something new, something different from what you've tried so far. Your former strategy was frowning all the time: How has that worked out for you?"

I might ask, "Would you rather be honestly trapped in a downward spiral of sadness and despair, or would you rather kick start those unfamiliar feelings of happiness and hope? Which direction would you like to go? The part that demands faux honesty is the part that is dragging you down."

One of my colleagues, upon reading an online discussion of laughter exercises, asked, "Isn't it all a bit silly?"

I replied, "Yes, it's wonderfully silly. But which is really more foolish: Deciding to laugh on purpose, taking control of your neurochemistry and the associated emotions, generating positive states at will—or continuing to be a slave to your emotions, letting either your internal ruminations or external forces control your happiness?"

Ultimately, I view hypnosis as a means for empowering my clients to take control of their lives, especially in areas that seemed beyond control. Unconditional Laughter is an excellent tool for claiming self-control. And there's nothing foolish about that.

Of course, as with any tool, I judge carefully what's right for the client in my office at the time. Some clients will want something very conventional; others want something very conversational. Some want a very fast solution; others want a slow, incremental change. Most can handle laughter as part of their hypnosis—even if it takes a little urging and explanation before they warm up to it—but a few simply can't allow themselves to laugh at their problems. As a hypnosis practitioner, it's my job to honor that, fitting the method to the client, not the client to the method. That doesn't devalue the tool.

For example, when I'm working with a client who has negative self-talk, I often ask them to hear that internal negativity in a silly, cartoonish voice. However, I had a very devout Catholic client who simply could not laugh at the voice of guilt within her head. That was out of the question for her. I asked how she would like to release those guilty thoughts, and she said that a church choir could sing them to God. Now, personally, I'd rather laugh—but her session was not about me. She listened to the church choir giving her guilt to God in song, and she got the relief she was seeking.

In the end, Laughnosis is a valuable tool to have in your belt. Remember that a screwdriver cannot drive a nail, nor can a hammer effectively drive a screw--yet both tools have their place.

EXERCISES

Exercise One: Stress Ball with Laughter

One of my favorite techniques is what I call "Stress Ball," and I've found that adding laughter to it simply turbo-charges the process, which goes like this:

1. Elicit a state of stress. (Words in italics are to be spoken)

Think about some obstacle in your life, something that causes stress. Close your eyes and really picture what you see when you are dealing with that obstacle. Perhaps it's a face or a location; maybe you think about the words that are said, or someone's annoying voice. Think of every detail related to that until you find yourself feeling some stress coming on.

2. Elicit submodalities.

Where do you feel it in your body?

What color is it?

What sound does it make?

3. Move stress to a shoulder.

Move that stress over to your shoulder—right shoulder if you're right-handed, left shoulder for left-handed. Picture the color there; hear the sound from there. You may feel some tightness. Let me know when it's there.

4. Shift stress to hand.

Move that stress down to the palm of your hand; picture it forming a ball.

At this point you can either instruct the client to hold the ball of stress in the palm of the hand, or you can request a fist at the end of a stiff, straight arm if you want to induce arm catalepsy as part of this process.

Let me know when all of the stress is in the hand.

5. Release the stress.

Now in a moment I will ask you to take a big, deep breath in. Then I'll count down from three to one before clapping my hands. When I clap my hands, you'll breathe out forcefully and shoot that ball of stress into outer space, letting the arm from the fingertips to the shoulder relax completely, falling at your side.

Breathe in. THREE, TWO, ONE! [Clap hands.]

Watch it go past the Earth's atmosphere, past the Earth's gravity, past the Moon, past the planets, past the stars, getting farther and farther away until finally it is sucked into a black hole or burnt up in a far away star and it is gone, gone, GONE!

6. Repeat.

Now, releasing stress is a bit like weeding a garden: After you get the big weeds, the smaller weeds are visible. So gather all those lesser stresses, move them to your shoulder, then move them to your hand. Let me know when they're there.

As before, you'll take a big deep breath in, I'll count down, and then you'll breathe out forcefully as you shoot the stress into outer space. Only this time, when you breathe out, please make a loud laughing noise with that breath. You don't have to feel like laughing, you can just make the noise as loud as you can.

Breathe in. THREE, TWO, ONE! [Clap and then make a laughing noise with your client.]

Watch it go past the Earth's atmosphere, past the Earth's gravity, past the Moon, past the planets, past the stars, getting farther and farther away. If any part tried to come back and bother you, it would burn up on re-entry, but you know once something is moving in space, it keeps getting farther and farther away until finally it is sucked into a black hole or burnt up in a far away star and it is gone, gone, GONE!

7. Repeat again.

By now you're becoming an expert at this, so you can notice the final weeds, the stresses that are barely poking through the surface but which might have deep roots. Pull those stresses up by the roots and move them to your shoulder and then your hand.

As before, you'll take a big deep breath in and laugh this stress into outer space. However, so that you'll take ownership of this process and use it whenever you need it, I want you to decide when you're ready to laugh away this obstacle. When you do, laugh so hard that you convince me you've just seen something hilarious.

[Wait for the client, but then join in the laughter.]

Watch it go past the Earth's atmosphere, past the Earth's gravity, past the Moon, past the planets, past the stars, getting farther and farther away. If any part tried to come back and bother you, it would burn up on re-entry, but you know once something is moving in space, all that stress, along with the ability to make more, keeps getting farther and farther away until finally it is sucked into a black hole or burnt up in a far away star and it is gone, gone, GONE!

8. Celebrate!

At this point, your client will probably be quite amazed at having released this problem, so congratulate them and ask for a high-five. I often ask at this point, "Where'd the stress go? It's gone!" or "Did you know your mind was this powerful?"

Notes:

Though I use stress as the example, this can be done with any unwelcome emotion or even an unwelcome habit.

Of course, you should vary the wording of this and all exercises presented in the book according to the situation.

Exercise Two: Laughter Bubble Plus

The Laughter Bubble is an exercise often used in Laughter Yoga, but it makes such a good follow-up to the Stress Ball that I want to include it here. Also, I'll be adding in a few hypnotic twists to the process.

1. Fill core with laughter.

Imagine that laughter has a color, and imagine that color, that "laughter energy," flowing into your body, filling it up. Maybe it flows into your feet from within the earth, or maybe into the top of your head from the stars, or maybe into your heart from the sun. The important thing is that there is an inexhaustible supply of laughter flowing into you. Start making laughing noises as you do this.

[If you've just done Stress Ball, emphasize the idea that this laughter is filling the spaces previously filled by stress, so that there's no room left for any negative emotion.]

2. Create Laughter Bubble.

Now keep laughing as you picture that light flowing up your spinal cord, spilling out at the top of your head, like water from a fountain, to flow down around you, forming a sphere, a bubble of laughter around you. When it gets to the ground, it gets pulled up into your body through the soles of your feet. With each breath in, it flows up through you; with each breath out, it flows down and around you. Keep laughing as it gets brighter.

3. Strengthen Laughter Bubble.

With each breath, your Laughter Bubble gets stronger, the light acting like an electromagnet that draws more joy and peace to you while repelling anything negative. In fact, it's so bright that no darkness may enter. Every time you breathe, it's strengthened, and every time you laugh, doubly so.

4. Practice Repelling Negativity.

In fact right now, I'm going to start cursing at you in gibberish. As I do, just keep laughing, imagining that all this negativity is sliding right off the bubble. The angrier I get, the more you laugh.

[Curse at your client in gibberish — nonsense sounds akin to made-up language. Sound angry. Shake your finger at them. Act increasingly frustrated, then resigned that your anger cannot penetrate their shield.]

5. OPTIONAL: Advanced Practice for Clients Ready to Handle It

Now, I'm going to switch out of gibberish, but you can find your bubble just gets stronger as you keep laughing.

[Actually say or shout shaming, hurtful things at your client as he or she continues to laugh. You will have to gauge this exercise carefully, making sure that you don't go beyond what your client can handle. Even though this may seem mean, it can be very liberating for your client to laugh at statements that previously produced shame.]

Exercise Three: Bi-LAUGHTER-al Stimulation

One technique used in hypnosis is bilateral stimulation—the activation of both brain-spheres in a rapid alternating pattern. Peter Brown, MD, in *The Hypnotic Brain,* discusses bilateral stimulation as a means of inducing trance, even mentioning that yogis practice breathing through alternate nostrils by blocking the airways with their thumbs. The therapeutic technique of *Eye Movement Desensitization and Reprogramming* (EMDR) uses bilateral stimulation, not just of the visual sense, but also the aural and kinesthetic senses. Though the founder of EMDR has insisted it is not hypnosis, it's hard to miss the similarity to the swinging pocket watch trance induction that has become iconic. Of course, students of Melissa Tiers' *Integrative Hypnosis* are familiar with her bilateral stimulation technique (also called "the ball toss").

Bi-laughter-al stimulation combines bilateral movement with Amy Cuddy's power pose research and, of course, the benefits of laughter. It's an excellent way to start the day; in fact, if I wake up and don't feel like getting out of bed, I do three rounds of bi-laughter-al stimulation with silent and initially half-hearted laughter. That's generally enough to get me going. It's a great exercise to perform during a morning shower. Bi-laughter-al stimulation can also be a great pick-me-up during a day at work, and it can even be modified to use while driving.

Here are the steps for Bi-LAUGHTER-al Stimulation:

1. Stand up with your feet shoulder-width apart, shoulders back, chest out, chin up, arms akimbo. This is a power pose known as "Standing like a Super-hero." (Of course, if you're in bed or driving, disregard the pose.)

2. Raise your eyebrows. Stretch your mouth into an exaggerated smile.

3. Place your hands on the outside of your thighs, and begin alternately patting each thigh.

4. In rhythm with the patting, make a simulated laughing noise that rhymes with "thigh": *high, high, high, high, high.*

5. Continuing the alternating rhythm, pat your belly while making a Santa-like laughing sound: *ho, ho, ho, ho, ho.*

6. Continuing the alternating rhythm, tap your chest in a Tarzan-like fashion: *ha, ha, ha, ha, ha.*

7. Continuing the alternating rhythm, gently tap the sides of your head, as though you were plotting something fiendish: *hee, hee, hee, hee, hee.*

8. Raise your hands above your head in a celebratory fashion: *woo, hoo, hoo, hoo, hoo!*

9. Repeat from step 3, increasing your speed each time.

Note: I find that I raise the pitch of my laughter slightly as I pat up the body.

Driving Modification

When on long drives or stuck in rush-hour slow-downs, I use a variant of this exercise to keep me alert but in good spirits. Of course, you should stay safe by focusing all of your attention on driving when road conditions warrant it.

Variant One: Keeping your left hand safely on the steering wheel, pat and laugh up the right side of the body. When you get to "woo-hoo," tap on the ceiling of your car. Then switch sides, keeping your right hand safely on the steering wheel while laughing your way up the left side of your body.

Variant Two: Keeping your left hand safely on the steering wheel, pat on your right thigh, laughing, "high, high, high." Then switch sides, keeping your right hand on the steering wheel while patting and laughing on the left thigh. Switch sides and work your way up the body in this fashion.

Bonus: When driving, I often cuss or express frustration at irritations that are not life-threatening and ultimately have minimal impact on my trip. I have started training myself to laugh immediately after cussing any time I'm driving—I'm actually laughing at how ridiculous it is to let a minimal setback affect my mood. The laughter is a way of taking back control.

Exercise Four: Laughter-Mations

We've all heard of affirmations, whether it's affirmations from a child's story:

"I think I can, I think I can."

Or from a parody self-help guru:

"I'm smart enough, I'm good enough, and dog gone it, people like me."

Or even the original affirmation:

"Everyday in every way, I'm getting better and better."

That last one was invented by Emile Coue, a hypnotist who realized that he didn't have to get clients into deep trance for suggestions to be effective. In fact, he would specifically say, "I'm not going to put you to sleep. There's no need." A big part of his method instructed people to simply repeat his famous affirmation over and over, as though they were praying the rosary.

The problem with affirmations is that their success is often hit-or-miss. If your lips are busy saying Yes to life, but your heart is saying, "Don't believe your lips," you basically have your critical faculty interfering with (and counter-acting) your affirmations. In fact, for some severely depressed people, repeating positive affirmations with the mouth just makes the depression shout louder on the inside.

One way around this is to use affirmations in a deep hypnotic trance, where they are called "Direct Suggestions." After all, deep trance bypasses the critical faculty. However, an easier and more fun way that you can bypass the critical faculty and implant self-suggestion is through Laughter-mation.

The trick to a Laughter-mation is to take any affirmations you want to use, and turn the words into laughter by inserting H-sounds in strategic locations:

"I luh-huh-huh-huv mysel-hel-hel-helf."

Of course, this will sound silly and may provoke spontaneous laughter. That silliness will distract you from the content of the statement, thus bypassing your mind's gatekeeper.

(Credit for inspiring this idea goes to Dave Berman, who invented a Laughter Yoga exercise called "Laughing around the World," in which participants turn various place names into laughs.)

Exercise Five: Body-Positive Laughter-Mations

Negative body image is a problem many people deal with, so this set of Laughter-mations helps foster a better relationship with one's body. They can be done in a sitting or standing position.

1. Feet.

Motion: Lift your toes and the balls of your feet, rapidly alternating your right and left feet.
Affirmation: "I love my fee-hee-hee-hee-hee-heet."
Repeat several times.

2. Thighs

Motion: Pat the outside of your thighs with your hands, rapidly alternating left and right.
Affirmation: "I love my thigh-high-high-high-high-highs."
Repeat several times.

3. Seat

Motion: Pat your butt cheeks, rapidly alternating left and right.
Affirmation: "I love my buh-huh-huh-huh-huh-hut."
Repeat several times.

4. Belly

Motion: Pat your belly, rapidly alternating left and right.
Affirmation: "I love my belly-hee-hee-hee-hee."
Repeat several times.

5. Chest

Motion: Pat your chest, rapidly alternating left and right.
Affirmation: "I love my cheh-heh-heh-heh-heh-hest."
Repeat several times.

6. Head

Motion: Tap the sides of head, rapidly alternating left and right.
Affirmation: "I love my heh-heh-heh-heh-head."
Repeat several times.

7. Body

Motion: Reach as high above your head as possible, wiggling hands
Affirmation: "I love my body-hee-hee-hee-hee."
Repeat several times.

Exercise Six: Laughter as an Auditory Submodality Shift

For those of you not into Neuro-Linguistic Programming (NLP), please forgive me for throwing around a bit of jargon. An auditory submodality is simply a parameter for describing a sound; for instance, a voice can be loud or quiet, high-pitched or low-pitched, slow or fast. A very effective NLP technique for dealing with negative self-talk is to actually change (or shift) the submodalities of a statement without changing the content. In other words, if you tend to think to yourself, "I'll never succeed," you can take the impact out of that statement by slowing it down in your mind, or speeding it up and making it ludicrously high-pitched.

A while back I ended up in a discussion on Facebook that got rather nasty. One of the participants was saying particularly hurtful things to me and those who agreed with me, and I found those insults reverberating in my mind, fanning the flames of my anger.

So, I took the statements and turned them into laughter. "You're a moron who doesn't get science" became:

"She said I'm a mo-ho-ho-ho-ra-ha-ha-ha-on who does-uh-uh-uh-uhn't ge-heh-heh-heh-hit sci-high-high-high-hience!"

I did this with several of the statements that had gotten under my skin, laughing them aloud, and I soon found that they no longer bothered me. In fact, thinking about the conversation, I found nothing but amusement.

I have long maintained that if you can be amused by idiots and ass-holes, you will never lack for entertainment.

So, for someone who is plagued with negative self-talk or who takes insults to heart, this is an excellent way to change one's thoughts.

Exercise Seven: Riddikulus Charm / Laughter Swish

Earlier in this book, I explained the NLP Swish Pattern, in which the participant ties a triggering image to a preferred response image, and I pointed out that many of the value-based exercises of Laughter Yoga follow a similar format. I want to expand on that, but I'd like to make a brief Harry Potter reference in the process.

In *Harry Potter and Prisoner of Azkaban,* the students of Hogwarts are taught a spell called "The Riddikulus Charm." Their teacher unleashes a Boggart, a monster that takes on the form of whatever scares its victim the most. To defeat the Boggart, each student waves a wand at the creature, shouting "Riddikulus" at it, whereupon the monster's appearance changes in some ridiculous and comical way, provoking laughter from the recently terrified child.

Now, I don't know if J.K. Rowling is familiar with NLP and/or Laughter Yoga, but the Riddikulus Charm is essentially a Visual Swish with laughter involved.

So in your office, when a client is confronted with a fear, one approach is to ask, "What would have to change about the appearance of this thing you were afraid of, in order for it to look so funny you would laugh at it?" For example, a client might say, "Well, if those bullies I remember all had enormous red clown noses, I'd have to laugh at them."

From that point, it's a simple matter to perform a Swish Pattern:

Now, picture those bullies who picked on you in fifth grade. Let that image get smaller and smaller, and then let it be suddenly replaced by the image of them with silly clown noses, getting bigger and bigger.

[If your client isn't laughing spontaneously, ask for a laughing noise.]

Now let the screen go blank. Picture those bullies who picked on you in fifth grade. Let that image get smaller and smaller, and then let it be suddenly replaced by the image of them with silly clown noses, getting bigger and bigger. Laugh!

[Repeat this process, faster and faster, until the client laughs or at least grins whenever thinking of those bullies.]

Exercise Eight: Laughter Re-Programming

All of us have things in our lives that we have to do but we don't necessarily enjoy. Maybe we do them, but the act produces anger or frustration every time.

For example, there was a husband who felt that part of doing any job was putting away the tools and the extra equipment when the job was done. So if he was going to make coffee for himself and his wife, he would make sure to put the bag of coffee beans back in the freezer when he was done. Even though it was a very minor thing, he felt frustrated any time his wife made coffee, because he would find the beans sitting out on the counter. He recognized that he'd be better off just appreciating that he had a loving wife who made coffee, but despite his attempts to be reasonable and enlightened about it, he found that putting away the coffee beans produced unwelcome anger and resentment—not a great way to start the day, nor a good way to sustain a happy marriage..

So, one day at Laughter Yoga class, the leader asked all the members to pantomime doing something they don't enjoy while simultaneously laughing enthusiastically. The husband in this story chose putting away the coffee beans. Since the exercise lasted several minutes, he repeated the pantomime (which inevitably involved visualizing the action as well) several times while laughing uproariously.

Much to his surprise, the next morning (and every morning since then), as he picked up the coffee beans to put them away, he started chuckling to himself. Although he didn't laugh uproariously, he did feel content and mildly happy instead of frustrated. In Pavlovian terms, the old stimulus (putting away the coffee beans) was now anchored to a new response (laughing or smiling, rather than feeling angry). In the hypnosis world, we call this collapsing anchors. He was quite pleased with his new programming.

Here is the process for enjoying what you can't change:

1. Identify something you have to do on a regular basis, but don't enjoy doing. When you've verified that it's not something you can avoid doing, recognize that the only thing that can change is your own reaction to it.

2. Close your eyes and imagine yourself in the place where you have to do that unpleasant task. Visualize the important things that are involved in the action. If any people are involved, picture them as well.

3. Pantomime performing the action and visualize yourself doing it as well. If it's necessary to open your eyes to safely pantomime, do so — you can still visualize with your eyes open.

4. Still pantomiming and visualizing, laugh enthusiastically. If you don't feel like laughing, make laughing noises. (Fake it 'till you make it.)

5. Continue the process for three to five minutes, or until you feel your mood lighten.

6. Repeat as needed.

Notes:

I have actually applied the Laughter Reprogramming technique with a client who had such an intense fear of spiders that he could not crush one in his house; instead, he would flee in terror. When all of the standard phobia removal techniques had barely made a dent, I asked him to simply visualize swatting a spider while making a laughing noise. We repeated this activity for around twenty minutes. When he got home that evening, as luck would have it, the first thing he saw was a spider on the wall. The first thing he did was smash it.

Exercise Nine: Laughter Re-Programming for Procrastination

Sometimes we want to do something, but we feel trapped in procrastination. This often occurs when we feel overwhelmed at all the steps needed to complete a big project, or when we have so many different tasks to do that we simply don't feel motivated to do any of them.

Fortunately, the Laughter Re-Programming process described in the previous section can help us out of being stuck. Here is the process:

1. Identify the end goal. Perhaps it's having a book published, or being in better shape, or just clearing all the projects off your desk. Whatever it is, for a brief moment, focus on the outcome—the top of the metaphorical mountain you feel you need to climb.

2. Close your eyes and let yourself be on the mountaintop. Really form and step into the image of your life as you accomplish your goal. Notice what you see, hear, feel, smell, taste, and think. Let it really sink in.

3. Now imagine grabbing that reality by the corners, compressing it into tiny seed, and planting that seed in the center of your heart.

4. Float back down to the present, still able to look at the mountain.

5. Identify one to three actions you can take in the next 24 hours to move yourself closer to the mountain.

6. Pick out one of those actions you are ready to do as soon as possible.

7. Pantomime and visualize yourself taking that action while laughing heartily. If it's necessary to open your eyes to safely pantomime, do so—you can still visualize with your eyes open. If you don't feel like laughing, make laughing noises, and you'll soon find yourself laughing spontaneously.

8. Continue for three to five minutes, or until you feel yourself compelled to take action.

9. When the task is done, repeat with each additional step that moves you closer to your goal.

Note: If there is some obstacle preventing you from taking the actions you identified, then you need to pick out three things that get you closer to removing that obstacle, and do this process with those things. It's all about baby steps.

Becoming Laughnotic

One of the best things about being a hypnotist is that you get to improvise and put your own spin on popular techniques. Good hypnosis trainers often speak of "being hypnotic" rather than "doing hypnosis."

The union of hypnosis and Unconditional Laughter is a fruitful one, and I can in no way lay exclusive claim to the concept of Laughnosis. The exercises and insights presented here arose from discussions I had with fellow practitioners, and it's my sincere hope that as a reader, you'll be inspired to find new and interesting ways to incorporate laughter in your sessions.

To spur your creativity further, I want to mention a few other ways my colleagues and I have thrown laughter into the hypnotic mix, especially for our clients suffering from Intense Chronic Seriosity:

Spin Technique: Many practitioners ask a client to identify a color, shape, location, and trajectory of an emotion, craving, or even physical pain — visualizing it as a spinning object. The next step is to picture moving the imagined object out of the body, reversing the spin (and possibly changing other aspects as well), and then placing the reversed object back in the body. Several years ago, brilliant hypnotist Melissa Tiers told me about spinning some laughter into the object before putting it back in the body. I've used this to great effect with clients, even nullifying severe OCD symptoms.

Circle of Excellence: This is a well-known NLP spatial anchoring technique in which the client steps into a visualized circle on the ground, building the desired state with appropriate colors, stances, words, gestures, memories, and role models. I will typically include stepping in and laughing uproariously as part of building the resource state.

Tapping and Laughing: For those fond of Emotional Freedom Technique (EFT), hypnosis author Kelley Woods has combined the tapping patterns of EFT with Unconditional Laughter. Though I'm not an EFT user, I like this variant as it removes any need for an affirmation to be remembered. Of course, tapping could easily be combined with Laughter-mations. (Tap and Laugh is described in more detail in *Laughter for the Health of It* by Dave Berman and Kelley Woods.)

Pain Train: Scott Sandland, founder of the Hypnosis Practitioner Training Institute, is famous for having his clients visualize being hit by a metaphorical train carrying everything they've ever run from, letting the train pass through them — and then hitting them with it twice more. Though not for the faint of heart, it's a surprisingly empowering experience. On the final pass, I sometimes instruct my clients to laugh loudly as the train dissolves.

Chakra Laughter: One of my Hindu clients asked me to help him visualize energy flowing through his chakras, and I was happy to help. After he'd practiced that for a few weeks, I invited him to move laughter energy through his chakras, tickling them until each one laughed. We even explored laughing the vowel sounds associated with each energy center.

Once you fully absorb the effectiveness of Unconditional Laughter as a tool for change, you'll find yourself becoming spontaneously laughnotic.

FINAL WORDS

Shoulders of Giants

While Laughnosis contains some innovations and variations that I can lay claim to as the products of my fevered imagination, I would be remiss if I didn't recognize that this work is only possible because of some amazing work that has gone before me.

First off, Madan Kataria, MD, collaborated with yoga teacher Madhuri Kataria to introduce Laughter Yoga to the world roughly twenty years before this writing. Perhaps the most brilliant innovation of Laughter Yoga is its focus on Unconditional Laughter — that is, laughter that occurs because we decide to laugh, as opposed to Conditional Laughter, which depends on jokes, comedy, humor, or some other external stimulus to make us laugh. I am proud to be a Certified Laughter Yoga Leader, and I'm indebted to the work of Dr. Kataria and the Laughter Yoga community at large.

Second, veteran hypnosis practitioner Michael Ellner pioneered the idea of hypnotists as "Hope Coaches," specialists in teaching the hopeless to foster states of optimism, enthusiasm, and bliss. He was the first person to point out to me the prevalence of Fun Deficiency (which I liken to Intense Chronic Seriosity).

More immediately, the exercises and insights in this book were catalyzed by discussions with my colleague and friend, Laughter Ambassador Dave Berman, who introduced me to the wonders of Laughter Yoga. He and Kelley T. Woods have written an excellent book called *Laughter for the Health of It,* which has a much more comprehensive survey of the therapeutic applications of Unconditional Laughter than the one I present here. I was privileged to serve as a sounding board for Dave while he and Kelley were writing, and I'm thankful they wrote a book that examines therapeutic laughter in great depth — thus saving me from having to cover the same ground.

I'd like to thank fellow hypnotist and author John McLean, whose brilliant book *Real Artists Ship* is a must read for anyone who wants to publish in the modern age.

Finally, I am indebted to April D. Porter for the lovely image used in the cover art.

References

Berman, Dave, and Woods, Kelley T. *Laughter for the Health of It.* 2015.

Kataria, Madan. *Laugh for No Reason.*

Maio, G.R., Olson, J.M., and Bush, J. "Telling Jokes that Disparage Social Groups: Effects on the Joke Tellers Stereotypes." *Journal of Applied Social Psychology* 27, no. 22 (1997): 1986-2000.

Seibt, B., and Forster, J. "Risky and Careful Processing under Stereotype Threat: How Regulatory Focus Can Enhance and Deteriorate Performance When Self Stereotypes are Active." *Journal of Personality and Social Psychology* 87 (2004): 38-56.

Carson, Shawn, and Marion, Jess. *The Swish: An In Depth Look at this Powerful NLP Pattern.* 2013.

Further Action

You're still here? I guess you like this book. Or you're a glutton for punishment. It's the first one, isn't it?

Because you've made it this far, I want to give you an important reminder: Don't make the mistake of thinking that laughter is only for your clients. Use these tools yourself and laugh loudly on a regular basis; it's an important part of self-care. No one is immune to Seriosity.

Because you have enjoyed reading about and applying these exercises in your own practice and your life, there are further steps you want to take:

First, find a Laughter Yoga group. There are free Laughter Clubs all around the world, and nothing quite compares to laughing with a group of like-minded strangers. A simple Internet search will help you find clubs near you. You may even be inspired to become a Certified Laughter Leader. If you can't join a group in person, there are phone and Skype laughter sessions happening almost any hour of the day; you'll find them easily with an Internet search.

Second, join Daily Laughers on FaceBook, YouTube, or Twitter. At the time of this writing (2016), Laughter Ambassador Dave Berman is creating a year-long series of Daily Laugh videos — so even if you can't make it to a club once a week, you can still laugh every day. Becoming a Daily Laugher will improve your life.

Third, share this book's message with others. Give it to your friends and clients; teach others the exercises. Go to Amazon and leave a five-star review talking about how much you love this book; you'll help me, but more importantly you'll help all those seeking an antidote to Seriosity.

(If you didn't enjoy the book, please don't tell anyone about it. Let it languish in obscurity!)

Made in the USA
Columbia, SC
13 April 2017